Q WHITE

LIVING YOUR BEST LIFE

Live a Happier, Healthier & Longer life in just 3 easy steps that take just 3 hours a week.

First edition

This book was professionally typeset on Reedsy.
Find out more at reedsy.com

Contents

1

Introduction

Hi, I'm Q White, this is me below with my beautiful family, I'm a real person just like you.

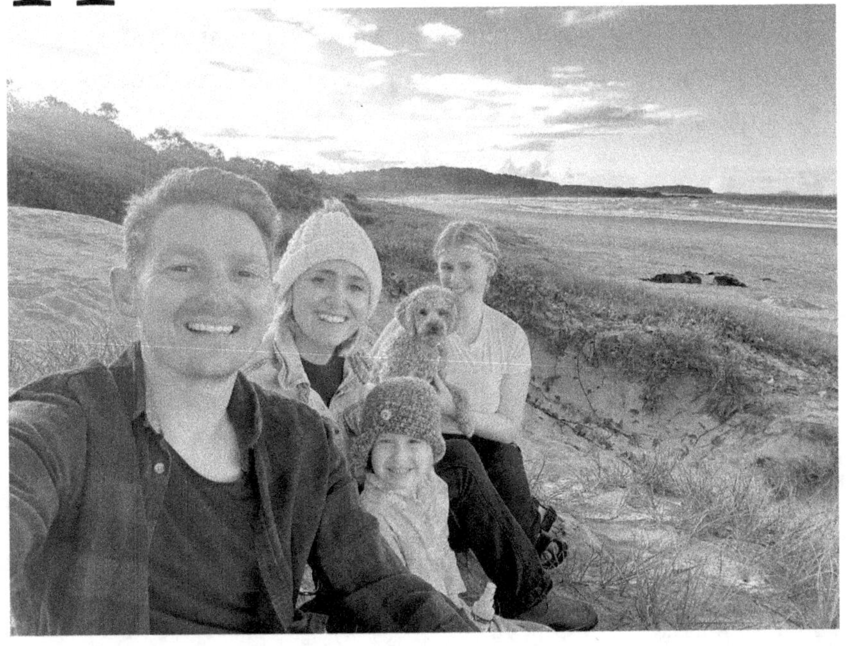

Life's been a whirlwind for me, full of challenges that often made it tough to focus on myself. I've dealt with gut health issues, managed the high stress and ups and downs of running a business, and raised two amazing daughters whilst trying to be the best husband I can be, all of which took a toll on my well-being. Remember the days when I hit the gym regularly? Those were the good old days!

So why did I write this book? Because I've been through the wringer and come out stronger. I live and breathe the concepts you'll read about every day, and I've spent thousands of hours researching, testing, and refining these ideas. I know there are many people out there just like me, struggling to find balance in a hectic world.

Here's the deal: life can be overwhelming, and it's easy to say no to new opportunities without even thinking. It's like our brains shut down before we get the chance to say yes. But this book is here to change that—it's your cheat code, your silver platter of info that makes it easy to start living your best life. No complicated stuff, just enough to get you going and make smarter choices for the long haul.

Let me share a little story with you. My 5-year-old daughter has been filling out her gratitude book almost every night for just over a year. Today, on May 30th, 2024, as I write this introduction, she looked up at me and said, "Isn't living just the best, Dad? Thank you so much for making it so awesome all the time!" It was one of those moments that make everything worthwhile.

The truth is, she's pretty much the one who named this book. While I often say "living the dream," she always tells me, "We're just living our best life, aren't we, Dad?" That's where the title came from—straight from the wisdom of a child who understands the power of gratitude and happiness.

Check out this photo of my daughter Luana, what do you see? I see complete contentment and I'm 100 percent committed to doing absolutely everything in my power to ensure she maintains that positive attitude towards life so that she can truly live her best life.

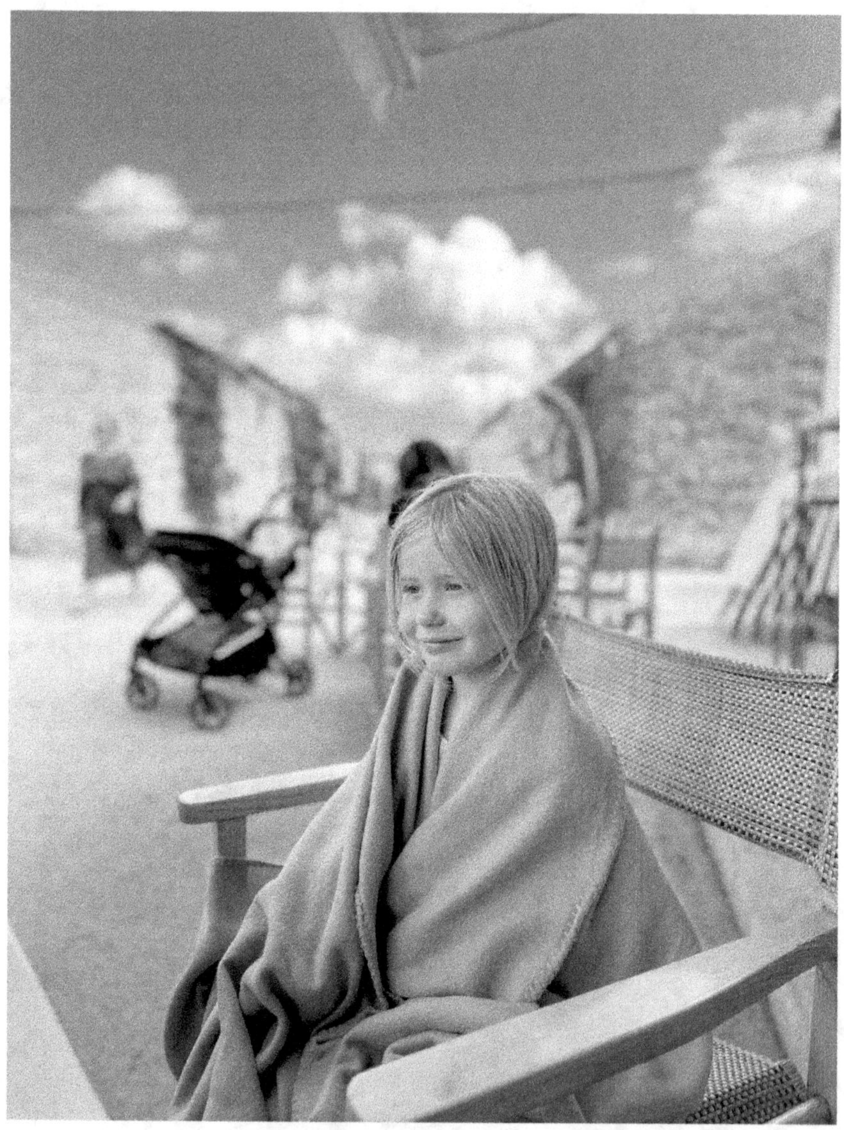

Let me share one more of Luana, while this photo was being taken she said the words "aah living our best life" I kid you not, right after she said "I'm getting some sun bro". Haha kids say the best stuff, right? We were on a boat on holiday in Italy so it certainly was a true statement at the time…

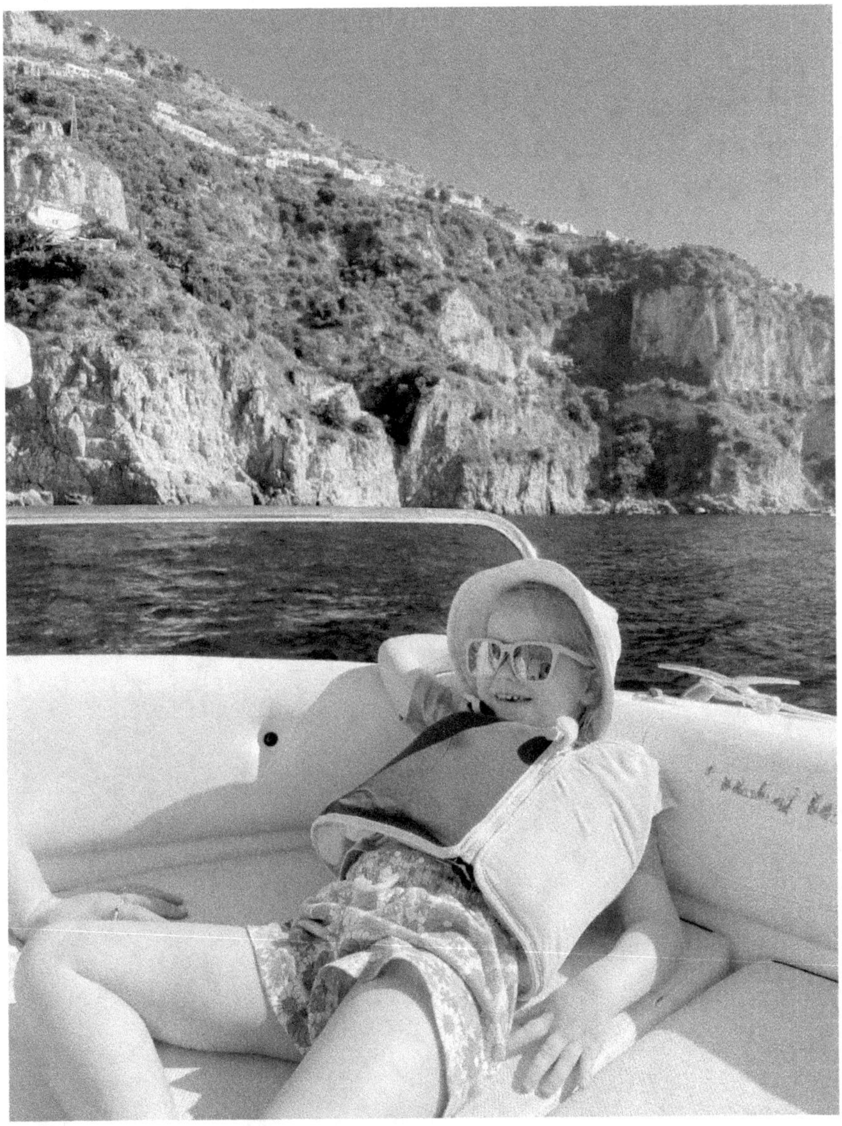

In this book, you'll find what I call the 'Mighty Triad Method' or, for short, the MTM —a simple yet powerful approach to integrating gratitude, exercise, and gut health into your routine. My goal is to make it easy and enjoyable for you to start building habits that lead to a happier, healthier life.

Before we get started, here's a short disclaimer: I am not a doctor, personal trainer, or dietitian. Everything you read in this book is not direct advice, but rather concepts and ideas for you to consider in making more informed decisions to improve your life. If you have any health concerns, please consult with a relevant specialist to ensure that following the concepts in this book does not cause any personal harm. Your health and safety are paramount, so always seek professional guidance when needed.

So, let's dive in and start living our best lives together. Cheers!

INTRODUCTION

2

Happy Hack: The Transformative Power of Practicing Gratitude for a Happier Life

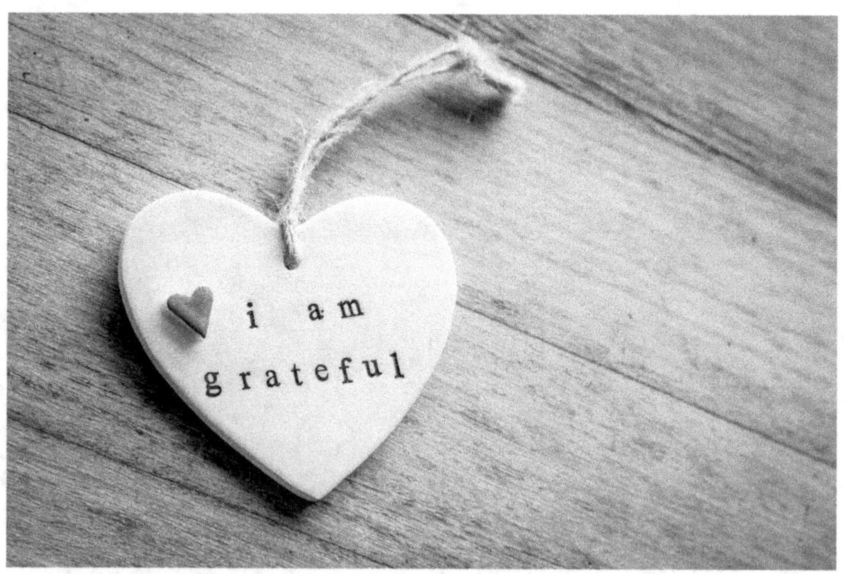

In today's world, anxiety and depression are skyrocketing, affecting millions of people. The pressures of modern life, combined with global crises, make mental health more important than ever. Amid these challenges, practicing gratitude stands out as a simple yet powerful tool to boost happiness and well-being. Spending just 10 minutes a day on gratitude can be a game-changer, offering profound benefits for both you and your loved ones.

The Crisis of Anxiety and Depression

Anxiety and depression rates are at an all-time high. According to the World Health Organization, depression is now the leading cause of disability worldwide, and anxiety disorders are the most common mental health issue globally. These conditions not only affect individuals but also ripple out to impact families, workplaces, and communities. Finding effective, accessible ways to enhance mental health is crucial in this environment.

Understanding Gratitude

Gratitude means recognizing and appreciating the positive aspects of life. It's about acknowledging the good things we often take for granted, from the kindness of others to simple daily pleasures. This mindful appreciation can shift our focus from what we lack to what we have, making us happier and more content.

The Mental Health Benefits of Gratitude

Research has shown that gratitude can significantly improve mental health. Studies by Dr. Robert Emmons and Dr. Michael McCullough have demonstrated that regular gratitude practice leads to higher levels of well-being and lower levels of depression and anxiety. Their research revealed that people who kept gratitude journals felt more optimistic and better about their lives overall compared to those who focused on negative or neutral life events.

Moreover, gratitude can enhance motivation in other areas of life, such as exercise and healthy eating. When we feel grateful, we're happier and more likely to take care of ourselves and pursue activities that boost our well-being. This holistic approach creates a positive feedback loop where feeling good encourages behaviors that enhance physical health, which in turn supports mental health.

How to Practice Gratitude

Incorporating gratitude into your daily routine is easy and doesn't take much time. Here are some fun and effective ways to practice gratitude for just 10 minutes a day:

1. Gratitude Journaling: Spend a few minutes each day writing down things you're grateful for. This practice shifts your focus from negative to positive experiences, helping to reframe your outlook on life.
2. Gratitude Meditation: Set aside time to meditate on the things you're thankful for. This can enhance your emotional resilience and reduce stress.
3. Expressing Gratitude: Take time to thank people in your life, whether through notes, calls, or in-person. This not only strengthens your relationships but also boosts your own happiness.

The Ripple Effect on Loved Ones

The benefits of practicing gratitude extend beyond yourself. When you cultivate a habit of gratitude, it positively impacts those around you. Expressing gratitude to family and friends can strengthen bonds, create a supportive environment, and improve overall relationship satisfaction. Kids, in particular, can learn from these practices, developing their own sense of gratitude and resilience.

Research shows that gratitude can enhance empathy and reduce aggression, making it easier to navigate conflicts and build stronger connections with others. This nurturing environment is crucial for the emotional development of children and the overall harmony of the household.

Conclusion

In a world where anxiety and depression are common, the practice of gratitude offers a powerful, accessible tool for improving mental health and fostering happiness. By dedicating just 10 minutes a day to gratitude exercises, you can transform your outlook on life, enhance your motivation to pursue healthy habits, and positively influence the well-being of those around you. Embrace the power of gratitude and watch it ripple through your life and the lives of your loved ones, creating a brighter, more fulfilling future for all.

One more note on gratitude: Think about everything you've just read and if you're a mother or a father, consider the impact you can have on your children by simply being a happier person yourself. That's powerful.

By integrating gratitude into your daily life, you can contribute to a global shift towards better mental health and deeper personal fulfillment.

3

Physical Health Hack: Easy, Long-Lasting Exercise Habits That Work

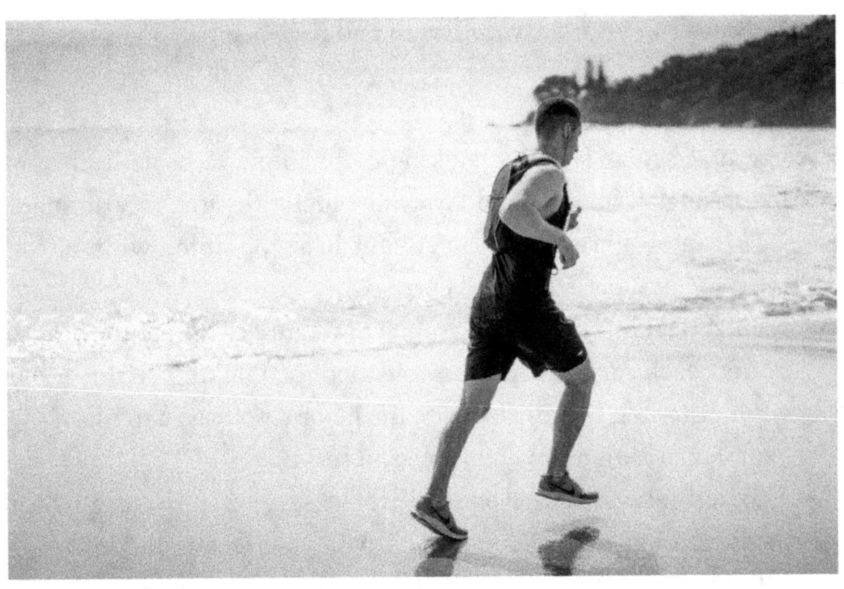

Creating sustainable exercise habits doesn't have to be a daunting task. With the right approach, you can integrate short, enjoyable activities into your daily routine that yield long-lasting and powerful benefits. This guide will show you how easy it is to develop such habits through activities like walking on the beach, practicing basic yoga techniques, and incorporating cold exposure and breathing exercises. Let's dive into these physical health hacks and how they can transform your life.

1. Walking on the Beach (or countryside, forest, or even in the city).

Walking is one of the simplest and most effective forms of exercise. When combined with the natural beauty and calming sounds of the beach, it becomes even more beneficial. Here's how a 30-minute walk on the beach can improve your health and well-being:

Benefits:

- Cardiovascular Health: Walking helps improve heart health by increasing circulation and lowering blood pressure. A 30-minute walk can be a great way to get your heart pumping without the intensity of more strenuous exercises.
- Mental Health: The soothing sound of waves and the natural beauty of the beach can reduce stress and anxiety. Walking on the beach while listening to your favorite music or a podcast can make the experience even more enjoyable and relaxing.
- Muscle Toning: Walking on sand provides natural resistance, which helps tone your muscles, particularly in your legs and core.
- Vitamin D: Exposure to sunlight while walking on the beach helps your body produce Vitamin D, essential for bone health and immune function.

How to Incorporate It:

- Schedule a 30-minute walk on the beach a few times a week.
- Use the time to listen to music, audiobooks, or podcasts to make the experience more enjoyable.
- Invite friends or family members to join you for added motivation and social interaction.

2. Basic Yoga Techniques

Yoga is an excellent way to improve flexibility, strength, and mental clarity. Practicing basic yoga techniques for just 15-20 minutes a day can have significant long-term benefits.

Benefits:

- Flexibility and Strength: Yoga helps improve flexibility and build muscle strength through various poses and stretches.
- Mental Clarity: Yoga promotes mindfulness and reduces stress through focused breathing and meditation practices.
- Balance and Posture: Regular yoga practice enhances balance and posture, which can prevent injuries and improve overall physical health.

How to Incorporate It:

- Follow online resources such as "Yoga by Adriene" on YouTube, which offers free, accessible yoga sessions for all levels.
- Set aside 15-20 minutes each day for your yoga practice. This could be in the morning to start your day or in the evening to wind down.
- Create a dedicated space for your yoga practice where you can focus without distractions.

3. The Power of Cold Showers and Ice Baths

Cold exposure through cold showers and ice baths is a powerful method for boosting physical and mental health. These practices, inspired by the Wim Hof Method, can have numerous benefits.

Benefits:

- Improved Circulation: Cold exposure stimulates blood flow, improving circulation and cardiovascular health.
- Boosted Immune System: Regular cold showers and ice baths can enhance your immune response, making you more resilient to illnesses.
- Reduced Inflammation: Cold exposure helps reduce inflammation and muscle soreness, aiding in recovery after exercise.
- Mental Resilience: The challenge of enduring cold temperatures can build mental toughness and resilience.

How to Incorporate It:

- Start with cold showers by gradually decreasing the water temperature at the end of your regular shower. Aim to stay under the cold water for at least 30 seconds, gradually increasing the duration as you become more comfortable.
- For ice baths, fill a tub with cold water and ice, and aim to stay submerged for a few minutes. Always consult with a healthcare provider before starting ice baths, especially if you have any health conditions.
- Combine cold exposure with deep breathing techniques from the Wim Hof Method to maximize the benefits.

4. Breathing Techniques Based on the Wim Hof Method

Breathing exercises are a cornerstone of the Wim Hof Method, known for their profound impact on physical and mental well-being.
Benefits:

- Enhanced Oxygen Intake: These techniques improve oxygen delivery to cells, boosting energy levels and physical performance.
- Stress Reduction: Controlled breathing activates the parasympathetic nervous system, reducing stress and promoting relaxation.
- Improved Focus and Clarity: Regular practice of breathing exercises can enhance mental focus and clarity, helping you stay centered and calm.

How to Incorporate It:

- Practice the Wim Hof breathing technique, which involves deep inhalations and exhalations followed by breath-holding phases. Start with a few rounds each morning to energize your day.
- Use these techniques during stressful situations to calm your mind and regain focus.
- Combine breathing exercises with your yoga practice or cold exposure sessions for a comprehensive approach to health and well-being.

Conclusion

Creating short, easy, and powerful exercise habits can have a lasting impact on your health and happiness. Whether it's a calming walk on the beach, a quick yoga session, or invigorating cold showers and breathing exercises, these practices can be seamlessly integrated into your daily routine.

By taking small steps towards these habits, you can transform not only your own life but also the lives of those around you.

Embrace these physical health hacks and watch how they make you happier, healthier, and more resilient in every aspect of your life.

4

Gut Health Hacks: Unlocking the Power of the Gut-Brain Connection

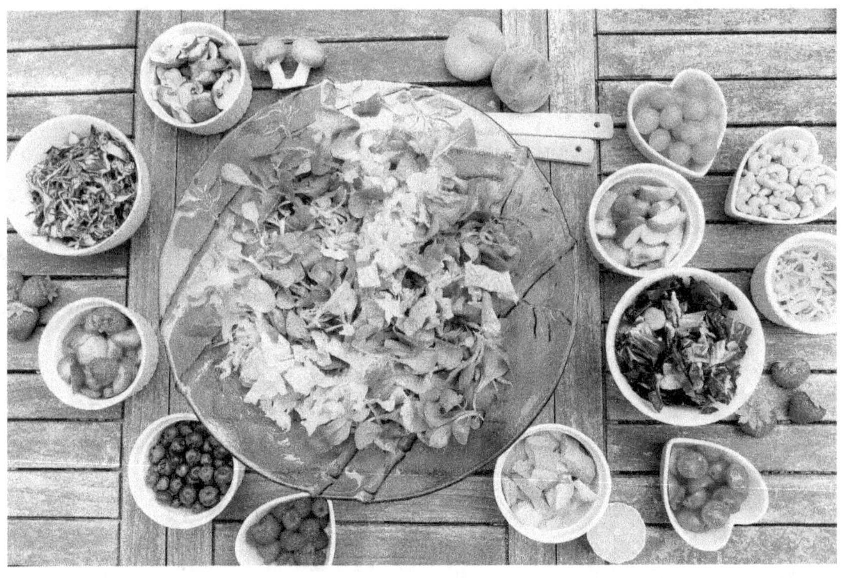

The gut-brain connection is one of the most fascinating areas of medical research today. As we continue to learn more about the gut's influence on our overall health, it becomes clear that a healthy gut is key to a healthy life. This guide will delve into the basics of gut health, explore its profound impact on our bodies, and provide practical tips on how to harness this knowledge through healthy eating habits.

The Gut-Brain Connection

The gut-brain axis is a complex communication network that links the emotional and cognitive centers of the brain with peripheral intestinal functions. This connection is primarily mediated by the gut microbiome, a diverse community of trillions of bacteria, viruses, and fungi living in our intestines.

The Role of Gut Microbes: Gut microbes play a crucial role in our health. They help digest food, produce vitamins, regulate the immune system, and protect against harmful bacteria. Notably, about 70% of our immune system resides in the gut, constantly interacting with gut microbes to maintain health and fend off disease.

Serotonin Production: Approximately 90% of the body's serotonin, often called the "happy hormone" because of its role in mood regulation, is produced in the gut. This indicates a direct link between gut health and mental well-being.

Impact on Hormones: Gut microbes can influence the production and regulation of various hormones, including estrogen and testosterone, which affect numerous bodily functions, from metabolism to reproductive health.

Benefits of a Healthy Gut

A well-balanced gut microbiome can have numerous benefits, including:

1. Improved Digestion: A healthy gut efficiently breaks down food and absorbs nutrients, reducing issues like bloating, constipation, and diarrhea.
2. Enhanced Immune Function: By maintaining a robust population of beneficial bacteria, a healthy gut can better protect against pathogens and reduce inflammation.
3. Better Mental Health: Given the significant production of serotonin in the gut, a healthy microbiome can improve mood and reduce symptoms of anxiety and depression.
4. Weight Management: Gut bacteria influence metabolism and fat storage. A balanced gut microbiome can help maintain a healthy weight.
5. Reduced Inflammation: Chronic inflammation is linked to numerous diseases, including heart disease, cancer, and diabetes. A healthy gut reduces inflammation, thereby lowering the risk of these illnesses.
6. Longevity: Healthy eating habits that support gut health are also associated with longer life spans. The concept of Blue Zones—regions where people live significantly longer—highlights diets rich in plant-based foods and low in processed foods, contributing to longevity and overall well-being .

Simple Hacks to Improve Gut Health

Improving gut health doesn't require expensive supplements or complicated routines. Here are some practical, food-based strategies inspired by Dr. Will Bulsiewicz's "Fiber Fueled" philosophy.

1. Eat More Fiber-Rich Foods: Fiber is the most important nutrient for gut health. It feeds the beneficial bacteria in the gut, promoting a diverse and balanced microbiome. Aim to include a variety of fruits, vegetables, whole grains, legumes, nuts, and seeds in your diet.Examples: Apples, bananas, berries, broccoli, carrots, lentils, quinoa, and almonds.

2. Incorporate Fermented Foods: Fermented foods are rich in probiotics, which are live beneficial bacteria. Including these foods in your diet can boost the population of good bacteria in your gut.Examples: Yogurt, kefir, sauerkraut, kimchi, miso, and kombucha.

3. Diversify Your Diet: A diverse diet leads to a diverse microbiome, which is associated with better gut health. Try to eat a wide range of plant-based foods to ensure you're getting various nutrients and fiber types.

4. Stay Hydrated: Water is essential for digestion and helps maintain the mucosal lining of the intestines, which supports the growth of beneficial bacteria.

5. Limit Processed Foods and Sugars: Processed foods and added sugars can disrupt the balance of bacteria in your gut, promoting the growth of harmful bacteria. Try to minimize your intake of these foods.

6. Shop Smart: Many grocery stores offer pre-prepared healthy options that can support gut health. Look for fresh soups and salads made from whole, plant-based ingredients. These can be convenient and nutritious choices for busy days.

Practical Tips for Daily Gut Health

Start Your Day with a Fiber-Packed Breakfast: Consider a smoothie made with fruits, vegetables, and a handful of nuts or seeds. This is an easy way to boost your fiber intake from the start of the day.

Snack Smart: Opt for fiber-rich snacks like an apple with almond butter or a handful of berries and nuts.

Make Lunch and Dinner Plant-Centric: Fill half your plate with vegetables, add a source of lean protein (like beans or lentils), and include a whole grain like brown rice or quinoa.

Experiment with Fermented Foods: If you're new to fermented foods, start with small portions and gradually increase. You might try adding a spoonful of sauerkraut to a salad or a serving of yogurt to your breakfast.

Shop for Convenience: Many supermarkets offer ready-to-eat healthy options such as pre-packaged salads, fresh vegetable soups, and snack packs of cut fruits and veggies. These can help you maintain a gut-friendly diet even on busy days.

Recipes to Get You Started

Gut-Friendly Smoothie:

- 1 banana
- 1 cup spinach
- 1/2 cup Greek yogurt
- 1 tablespoon chia seeds
- 1 cup almond milk
- Blend all ingredients until smooth.

Quinoa Salad with Mixed Vegetables:

- 1 cup cooked quinoa
- 1/2 cup chopped cucumber
- 1/2 cup cherry tomatoes, halved
- 1/4 cup red onion, diced
- 1/4 cup feta cheese
- 2 tablespoons olive oil
- 1 tablespoon lemon juice
- Salt and pepper to taste
- Mix all ingredients in a bowl and serve.

The Long-Term Impact

By incorporating these simple, plant-based strategies into your daily routine, you can significantly improve your gut health. Not only will you notice benefits like better digestion and increased energy, but you'll also be supporting your mental health and overall well-being. Furthermore, healthy gut habits are linked to a longer life, as evidenced by the dietary practices in Blue Zones, where people often live healthier, longer lives .

One final thought: if you're a parent, consider the impact of your gut health on your family. By prioritizing a healthy gut, you set a positive example for your children, encouraging them to adopt these beneficial habits. A healthy gut can lead to a happier, more vibrant life for you and your loved ones.

5

The Mighty Triad Method Health Hack: Integrating Gratitude, Physical Exercise, and Gut Health

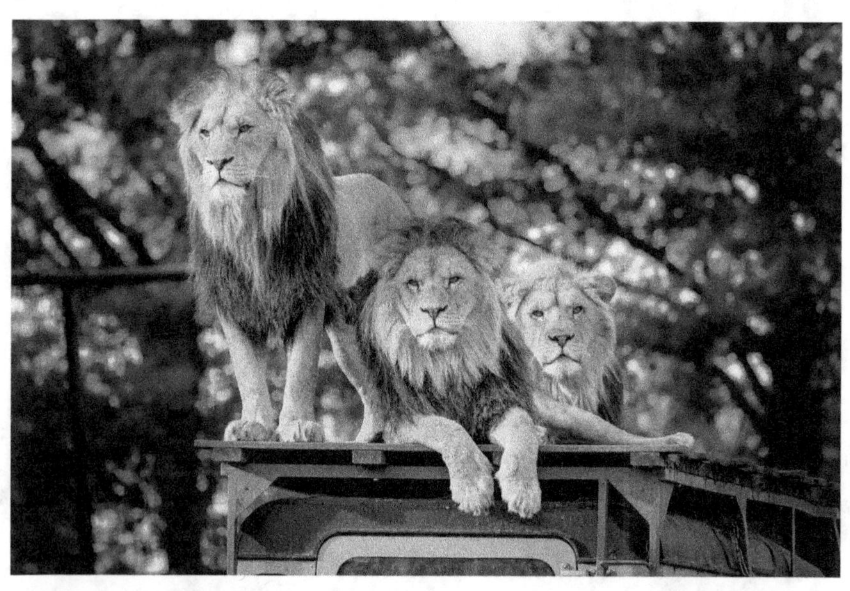

In the pursuit of a healthier, happier life, we often focus on individual strategies without recognizing how these practices can complement and enhance one another. By combining the transformative power of gratitude, the benefits of consistent physical exercise, and the foundational impact of gut health, we can create a synergistic approach that amplifies the effects of each component. Let's explore how these three hacks—practicing gratitude, engaging in regular physical activity, and maintaining gut health—interconnect and form the 'Mighty Triad Method' health hack.

1. The Transformative Power of Practicing Gratitude

Gratitude is more than just a feel-good emotion; it's a powerful practice that can reshape our mental landscape and overall well-being. Regularly practicing gratitude can significantly reduce symptoms of anxiety and depression, leading to a happier and more content life . This positive mental state can motivate us to engage in other health-promoting behaviors, such as exercise and healthy eating.

Impact on Physical Health: When we feel grateful, we are more likely to take care of our bodies. Gratitude can enhance our motivation to stay active, as it fosters a positive mindset and encourages us to prioritize our well-being . Engaging in physical activities, in turn, boosts our mood through the release of endorphins and other neurotransmitters, creating a positive feedback loop.

Connection to Gut Health: The practice of gratitude can reduce stress levels, which is beneficial for gut health. Chronic stress can negatively impact the gut microbiome, leading to digestive issues and inflammation . By reducing stress through gratitude, we create a more favorable environment for our gut bacteria, supporting overall health.

2. Easy, Long-Lasting Exercise Habits That Work

Regular physical exercise is crucial for maintaining physical health, mental well-being, and longevity. Simple habits like walking on the beach, practicing basic yoga techniques, and incorporating cold showers or ice baths can have profound effects on our health.

Mental Health Benefits: Exercise is a well-known mood enhancer. Activities like walking and yoga release endorphins, reduce anxiety, and improve sleep quality. These mental health benefits complement the positive effects of gratitude, creating a robust defense against stress and depression.

Support for Gut Health: Exercise also plays a significant role in gut health. Physical activity increases the diversity of gut bacteria, promotes healthy digestion, and reduces inflammation. A healthy gut, in turn, supports overall physical performance and recovery, making it easier to maintain an active lifestyle.

3. Unlocking the Power of the Gut-Brain Connection

Gut health is foundational to overall well-being. The gut-brain axis, a communication network linking the gut and the brain, underscores the importance of a healthy gut in regulating mood, immune function, and overall health.

Mental Health Benefits: A healthy gut produces neurotransmitters like serotonin, which influence mood and emotional well-being. By maintaining a balanced gut microbiome through a fiber-rich diet, fermented foods, and proper hydration, we support our mental health and enhance the effects of gratitude practices.

Enhancement of Physical Performance: Gut health directly impacts physical performance by optimizing nutrient absorption and reducing inflammation. When our gut is healthy, we have more energy and better stamina, which makes it easier to stay committed to our exercise routines.

The Synergistic Effect: The Mighty Triad Method Health Hack

By integrating gratitude, physical exercise, and gut health into our daily routines, we create a powerful synergy that enhances each component's benefits:

Enhanced Motivation and Adherence: Practicing gratitude can increase our motivation to exercise and eat healthily. When we feel grateful and positive, we are more likely to engage in activities that further boost our well-being.

Reduced Inflammation and Improved Recovery: Regular exercise and a healthy gut both contribute to reduced inflammation, which is crucial for preventing chronic diseases and supporting recovery after physical activity. This allows us to maintain an active lifestyle with less risk of injury and illness.

Improved Mental and Emotional Health: The combined effects of gratitude, exercise, and gut health create a robust framework for mental and emotional well-being. By reducing stress, enhancing mood, and promoting better sleep, we build a resilient foundation for a happier life.

Longevity and Quality of Life: Integrating these practices can contribute to a longer, healthier life. Healthy eating habits that support gut health are linked to increased longevity, as seen in the Blue Zones, regions where people live significantly longer due to their diets and lifestyles. Regular exercise and a positive mindset further enhance life quality and lifespan.

6

Implementing the Mighty Triad Method Health Hack in Just 3 Hours Per Week

Transforming your life through gratitude, exercise, and gut health might sound like a significant time commitment, but you can make profound changes with as little as three hours per week. By dedicating just one hour a day, three days a week, you can integrate these powerful health practices into your routine. Here's how to structure your week to maximize the benefits and set yourself on a path to a healthier, happier life.

The Mighty Triad Method Plan: Structure and Implementation

Each day's dedication consists of:

- 10 minutes of gratitude journaling: Reflect on and write about things you are grateful for to foster a positive mindset.
- 20 minutes of yoga or a brisk walk/jog: Engage in physical activity to boost mood and energy levels. Listening to your favorite music

30

during walks or jogs can enhance the experience.

- Cold exposure: Conclude your exercise with a cold shower, a swim in a river or the ocean, or an ice bath to invigorate and reduce inflammation.
- Healthy breakfast: Nourish your body with a nutritious, fiber-rich meal to support gut health and provide sustained energy for the day.

Here's a practical plan to follow:

Day 1: Morning Gratitude, Exercise, and Cold Exposure

- Gratitude (10 minutes): Start your day by writing in your gratitude journal. Reflect on three things you're thankful for and why they matter to you. This practice helps cultivate a positive outlook and reduces stress.
- Exercise (20 minutes): Engage in a brisk walk or jog, ideally in a natural setting like the beach or a park. Listen to your favorite music or a motivational podcast to enhance your experience.
- Cold Exposure (10 minutes): Finish your session with a cold shower, swim in a nearby river or ocean, or an ice bath. Cold exposure can reduce inflammation, boost mood, and increase overall energy levels.
- Healthy Breakfast (20 minutes): Prepare a fiber-rich breakfast, such as a smoothie with spinach, bananas, chia seeds, and almond milk, or oatmeal topped with berries and nuts. This meal will support your gut microbiome and provide sustained energy.

Day 2: Yoga, Cold Exposure, and Gut Health

- Gratitude (10 minutes): Begin with your gratitude journaling to foster a positive mindset for the day.
- Exercise (20 minutes): Follow along with a Yoga with Adriene video for a calming yet invigorating session. Yoga helps improve flexibility, strength, and mental clarity.
- Cold Exposure (10 minutes): After your yoga session, take a cold shower, swim, or ice bath to refresh and energize your body.
- Healthy Breakfast (20 minutes): Enjoy a gut-friendly meal like avocado toast with whole-grain bread, a side of fresh fruit, and a cup of green tea. This meal provides essential nutrients and supports digestive health.

Day 3: Mindful Walking, Cold Exposure, and Healthy Breakfast

- Gratitude (10 minutes): Start your day with gratitude journaling. Reflect on positive experiences and achievements, no matter how small.
- Exercise (20 minutes): Go for a brisk walk, focusing on mindfulness. Pay attention to your surroundings, your breath, and the sensations in your body. Listen to your favorite music to enhance your walk.
- Cold Exposure (10 minutes): Follow your walk with a cold shower, a swim in a natural body of water, or an ice bath to invigorate your senses and reduce inflammation.
- Healthy Breakfast (20 minutes): Prepare a nutritious breakfast like a quinoa bowl with mixed vegetables and a boiled egg, or a yogurt parfait with granola and fresh berries. This meal will fuel your body and support gut health.

The Benefits of Early Morning Exercise

Integrating early morning exercise into your routine can have profound impacts on your day and overall well-being:

1. Boosted Energy Levels: Morning exercise helps wake you up and gets your blood flowing, providing a natural energy boost that can last throughout the day. It helps you feel more alert and ready to tackle daily tasks.
2. Improved Mood: Physical activity triggers the release of endorphins, which are natural mood enhancers. Starting your day with exercise can set a positive tone, reducing stress and anxiety levels.
3. Enhanced Focus and Productivity: Exercise increases blood flow to the brain, which can improve cognitive function and concentration. This can lead to better performance at work or in other daily activities.
4. Consistent Routine: Exercising in the morning ensures that you get your workout done before the demands of the day interfere. It establishes a consistent routine, making it easier to stick to your fitness goals.

Practical Tips for Success

Prepare the Night Before: Lay out your exercise clothes and prepare any equipment or resources you'll need. This reduces the barriers to getting started in the morning.

Keep It Simple: Choose exercises and gratitude practices that you enjoy and that are easy to implement. This increases the likelihood that you'll stick with them.

Track Your Progress: Use a journal or an app to track your gratitude reflections, exercise routines, and eating habits. Seeing your progress can be motivating and help you stay on track.

Be Flexible: While consistency is important, it's also crucial to be flexible and adaptable. If you miss a session, don't get discouraged. Simply pick up where you left off.

Involve Others: Share your goals with friends or family members, or join a community of like-minded individuals. Having a support system can provide encouragement and accountability.

Profound Impact on Your Life

By dedicating just three hours a week to this integrated approach, you can experience significant improvements in your overall health and well-being:

Physical Health: Regular exercise and a healthy gut contribute to improved digestion, enhanced immune function, and reduced inflammation, which can lower the risk of chronic diseases.

Mental Health: Gratitude and physical activity together enhance mood, reduce stress, and improve sleep quality, fostering a more positive and resilient mindset.

Longevity and Quality of Life: Consistent healthy habits are linked to increased longevity and a higher quality of life. By nurturing your mind, body, and gut, you create a solid foundation for long-term health.

Daily Inspiration and Motivation: Starting your day with gratitude and exercise can inspire you to make healthier choices throughout the day. It sets a proactive tone, encouraging you to take on challenges with a positive attitude and greater energy.

Action Steps, for right now

1. Buy a gratitude journal online, there are 100's to choose from on Ebay, dont worry too much about which one you get, the important thing is that you just get one.
2. Open up the calendar app on your phone or computer and lock in 1 hour a day for 3 days (preferably early mornings) and add an event called ***MTM Live My Best Life*** and set it to repeat every week.
3. Go to the **Yoga with Adriene** Youtube channel and subscribe.
4. Find and save three breakfasts and three other meal recipes that you know you can commit to and make easily (set yourself up for success) that are packed with a diversity of fresh products that promotes gut health. I recommend using the Blue Zones recipes, you can find them here: https://www.bluezones.com/recipes/ and if you want to spend a little more time getting into healthy gut eating then I suggest reading **The Plant Fed Gut** by Dr. Will Bulsiewicz, you can find this on Amazon.
5. Go to your local supermarket and find some already made meals such as greek salads and/or, my favorite I get every week are fresh soups from the cold section and add a slice or two of sourdough if you want to make it a heavier meal. Add these into your weekly routine to help make eating fresh healthy meals a long lasting habit.

6. Say out loud right now: "I will commit to the MTM action steps and become a better version of myself and live my best life".

7

Conclusion

Wrapping things up, diving into the Mighty Triad Method Health Hack doesn't demand much time, but boy, does it pay off big time. Just set aside an hour a day, three days a week, and boom—you're on your way to weaving gratitude, exercise, and gut health into your everyday routine. This trio works like magic, boosting not just your physical and mental health, but also fueling a can-do attitude that sticks around for the long haul.

Now, here's the secret sauce: consistency and fun. Stick with activities that you actually enjoy, and keep at it regularly. Trust me, the more you stick with it, the easier it gets. These health hacks aren't just a one-time fix; they're lifelong companions on your journey to a better you.

As you embark on this journey, remember that your actions speak louder than words. By embracing these practices, you're not just transforming your own life—you're inspiring others to do the same.

And hey, let me share a little insider scoop: this book isn't just a book for me, It's a stepping stone. I've lived and breathed every word in these pages, and now, I'm gearing up to dive even deeper. More books, online courses—you name it. My mission? To equip folks like you with the tools, knowledge, and motivation they need to live their absolute best lives.

If you would like to be kept in the loop with all up and coming MTM news head to **themightytriadmethod.com and hit the subscribe button.**

If you have enjoyed this book please take just 2 minutes of your time to leave me a favorable review on Amazon as this will help me continue my mission to help as many people as possible to live their best lives.

So here's to you, here's to me, and here's to the journey ahead. Let's make every day count. Cheers!

Q White.

8

Resources

Publications – Gratitude works. (2011). Gratitude Works. Retrieved June 3, 2024, from http://emmons.faculty.ucdavis.edu/publications/

Gratitude Journal (Greater Good in Action). (2024, March 18). Greater Good Science Center. Retrieved June 3, 2024, from https://ggia.berkeley.edu/practice/gratitude_journal

MSc, E. S. (2019, February 4). The science and research on gratitude and happiness. PositivePsychology.com. Retrieved June 3, 2024, from https://positivepsychology.com/gratitude-happiness-research/

Wim Hof Method. (n.d.). Wim Hof Method. Retrieved June 3, 2024, from https://www.wimhofmethod.com/

The Plant Fed Gut, Empower Your Health, Dr. Will Bulsiewicz. (2020, September 8). Book - The Plant Fed Gut | Empower Your Health | Dr. Will

Bulsiewicz. Dr. Will Bulsiewicz | the Gut Health MD. Retrieved June 3, 2024, from https://theplantfedgut.com/book/

The Plant Fed Gut, Empower Your Health, Dr. Will Bulsiewicz. (2020b, November 19). *Research - The Plant Fed Gut | Empower Your Health | Dr. Will Bulsiewicz*. Dr. Will Bulsiewicz | the Gut Health MD. Retrieved June 3, 2024, from https://theplantfedgut.com/research/

Admin. (2023, November 17). *Recipes*. Blue Zones. Retrieved June 3, 2024, from https://www.bluezones.com/recipes/